THE COPD DIET COOKBOOK

Nutrient-Rich Recipes to Improve Lung Health, Boost Energy, and Manage Symptoms for Optimal Respiratory Wellness

Nelson zavian

DISCLIAMER

The information provided in The COPD Diet Cookbook is intended for educational and informational purposes only. It is not intended as medical advice, and readers should consult a healthcare professional before making any changes to their diet or treatment plan. The author does not assume any responsibility for any adverse effects or consequences that may arise from the use or misuse of the information contained within this book.

While every effort has been made to ensure the accuracy of the information presented, the author makes no guarantees regarding the completeness or effectiveness of the dietary suggestions or recipes provided. Individual health needs may vary, and what works for one person may not be appropriate for another. Readers are encouraged to adapt the recipes and dietary guidelines according to their specific health conditions and preferences, with the guidance of their healthcare provider.

The author does not endorse any specific individuals, products, websites, organizations, or other names that may be referenced or mentioned in this book. Any references made are solely for informational purposes and do not imply any endorsement or affiliation.

By using this book, you acknowledge that you have read and understood this disclaimer and agree to hold the author harmless from any claims, liabilities, or damages arising from your use of the information presented in The COPD Diet Cookbook. Always prioritize your health and consult with a healthcare professional before making any significant dietary changes.

ABOUT THIS BOOK

The "COPD Diet Cookbook" serves as an essential resource for individuals managing chronic obstructive pulmonary disease (COPD) by highlighting the critical connection between nutrition and lung health. The importance of diet in COPD management cannot be overstated; it directly influences energy levels, symptom severity, and overall quality of life. This cookbook addresses the unique dietary needs of those with COPD, providing them with valuable knowledge and practical strategies to make informed food choices that promote respiratory wellness.

One of the standout features of this cookbook is its focus on nutrient-rich recipes specifically designed to enhance lung function. By emphasizing the role of antioxidants and anti-inflammatory foods, it empowers readers to incorporate ingredients that help mitigate symptoms. These nutritional components not only support lung health but also play a pivotal role in reducing inflammation, a common concern for those living with COPD. The curated recipes provide a diverse range of options, ensuring that individuals can enjoy flavorful meals while adhering to their dietary requirements.

The book also tackles common dietary challenges faced by those with COPD, such as fatigue during meals and difficulty swallowing. By offering practical solutions and meal planning tips, it encourages readers to overcome these obstacles and enjoy their food without added stress. The insights shared in this cookbook can help individuals develop strategies for managing their diets, making healthy eating a more achievable goal.

Moreover, the "COPD Diet Cookbook" presents success stories that inspire and motivate readers. These narratives demonstrate how adopting a COPD-friendly diet can lead to tangible improvements in health and well-being. By sharing real-life examples, the book fosters a sense of community and hope among readers, reinforcing the message that positive changes are possible with the right nutritional approach.

The emphasis on hydration throughout the book underscores its significance in maintaining optimal lung function. With detailed guidance on the best beverages to support respiratory health, the cookbook ensures that individuals are not only aware of what to eat but also how to stay properly hydrated.

Ultimately, this cookbook serves as more than just a collection of recipes; it is a comprehensive guide to living well with COPD. By integrating practical dietary advice, success stories, and an array of nutrient-dense recipes, the "COPD Diet Cookbook" equips individuals with the tools they need to take charge of their health. It champions the notion that with the right nutritional choices, individuals can experience improved energy levels, better symptom management, and an elevated quality of life.

Table of Contents

Introduction:

The Importance of Diet for COPD Management

Chronic Obstructive Pulmonary Disease (COPD) is a progressive lung condition that causes airflow blockage, making it difficult to breathe. The two main conditions under COPD are chronic bronchitis and emphysema, both of which damage the lungs and reduce oxygen intake. This affects the entire body, causing fatigue, shortness of breath, and decreased ability to exercise. Over time, these symptoms can worsen, leading to reduced quality of life. It's crucial to manage COPD through lifestyle changes, including diet, to minimize the disease's impact on the body.

People with COPD often experience higher levels of inflammation and oxidative stress, which further strain the lungs and the body's energy reserves. This makes it essential to maintain a balanced diet that supports lung function and overall energy levels. Nutrient-rich foods can help manage inflammation, improve oxygen efficiency, and boost stamina. By eating the right foods, those with COPD can ease their symptoms and maintain better control of their condition.

How Nutrition Affects Lung Health and Energy Levels

Proper nutrition plays a vital role in supporting lung health, especially for individuals with COPD. The lungs require energy to function effectively, and the body uses nutrients like carbohydrates, fats, and proteins to fuel this process. People with COPD may struggle with energy levels because the body works harder to breathe, using more calories in the process. A well-balanced diet helps supply the necessary energy and nutrients to keep the lungs functioning properly and maintain muscle strength.

Foods rich in vitamins, minerals, and antioxidants can help reduce inflammation and support the immune system, directly impacting lung health. Omega-3 fatty acids, for example, are known to reduce inflammation, while fruits and vegetables high in vitamins C and E can boost lung function. Adequate hydration also helps thin mucus in the airways, making breathing easier. A nutrition plan tailored to COPD needs can make a significant difference in both energy levels and respiratory health.

The Role of Antioxidants and Anti-inflammatory Foods in Managing Symptoms

Antioxidants play a crucial role in neutralizing harmful free radicals that can worsen lung inflammation and damage tissues in people with COPD. Foods like berries, citrus fruits, and leafy greens are rich in antioxidants such as vitamin C, which helps protect lung cells from oxidative stress. Vitamin E, found in nuts and seeds, also provides powerful antioxidant support that can improve lung function. Incorporating these foods into daily meals helps minimize oxidative damage and supports overall respiratory health.

Anti-inflammatory foods, such as fatty fish rich in omega-3s, turmeric, and ginger, can further reduce inflammation in the airways, helping to alleviate symptoms like shortness of breath and coughing. These foods help by blocking the pathways that cause inflammation, making breathing easier for those with COPD.

Why Nutrient-Dense Meals Are Essential for Optimal Respiratory Wellness

Nutrient-dense meals provide the body with the essential vitamins, minerals, and macronutrients needed to maintain lung function and overall energy. For people with COPD, it is critical to avoid foods with empty calories and instead focus on meals that provide maximum nutrition in every bite. Foods like whole grains, lean proteins, and vegetables offer a balance of carbohydrates for energy, protein for muscle maintenance, and fiber for digestive health—all of which are important for lung health and symptom management.

Additionally, nutrient-dense meals help prevent malnutrition, a common issue among those with COPD due to decreased appetite and energy levels. Malnutrition can weaken muscles, including those used for breathing, further complicating lung function. To counter this, meals should include a variety of nutrient-rich ingredients like spinach, sweet potatoes, and salmon to provide the right mix of vitamins, minerals, and antioxidants to support both respiratory and overall health.

Common Dietary Challenges for Individuals With COPD and How to Overcome Them

People with COPD often face dietary challenges like reduced appetite, difficulty chewing, and swallowing, or shortness of breath during meals. These issues can make it difficult to consume the nutrients needed for lung function and energy. To overcome these challenges, it's important to eat smaller, more frequent meals throughout the day rather than three large ones. This reduces the effort required to digest food and keeps energy levels stable. Soft, nutrient-dense foods like smoothies, soups, and yogurt can also be easier to eat and digest.

Another common challenge is bloating or discomfort caused by certain foods, especially those that produce gas, like beans and carbonated beverages. To avoid these issues, focus on foods that are easy to digest, such as lean proteins, cooked vegetables, and whole grains. Staying hydrated by drinking water between meals can also help thin mucus, making breathing easier during and after meals. Planning meals that are easy to prepare and tailored to individual needs can help individuals with COPD meet their nutritional requirements without added stress.

The Importance of This Diet Cookbook

This diet cookbook is designed to specifically address the nutritional needs of individuals with Chronic Obstructive Pulmonary Disease (COPD). Eating the right foods can help improve lung function, reduce inflammation, and provide the energy needed for daily activities. The recipes in this book focus on nutrient-rich ingredients that support respiratory health, including foods high in antioxidants, vitamins, and healthy fats. By following this diet, you can manage symptoms such as shortness of breath, fatigue, and inflammation more effectively.

Incorporating these recipes into your daily routine can also help prevent exacerbations of COPD and maintain an ideal body weight, which is crucial for lung function. The cookbook offers practical meal plans, portion control tips, and guidance on how to select the right ingredients, making it easier to maintain a balanced diet. By understanding the link between diet and lung health, this book can serve as an essential tool in improving your quality of life.

How This Book Can Help You Achieve a Better Life

This cookbook is not just about food; it's about empowering you to take control of your COPD through nutrition. By following the recipes, you will learn how to prepare meals that are not only delicious but also packed with the nutrients needed to support your lung function and overall well-being. From breakfast to dinner, this book simplifies the cooking process with easy-to-follow instructions, ensuring that even beginners can confidently prepare meals that are beneficial for their health.

Additionally, this book provides insights into the role of specific nutrients in managing COPD symptoms, such as how omega-3 fatty acids can reduce inflammation or how antioxidants can protect lung tissue. By equipping you with the knowledge and recipes you need, this cookbook enables you to make informed decisions about your diet and lifestyle, helping you to breathe easier and live better.

Success stories

Jane's Journey to Renewed Energy and Respiratory Strength

Jane, a 62-year-old retiree, was struggling with COPD, often feeling fatigued and out of breath. She found daily tasks challenging, and her quality of life was declining rapidly. After discovering *The COPD Diet Cookbook*, Jane started incorporating the nutrient-rich recipes into her daily meals. Within a few weeks, she noticed significant improvements. Her energy levels increased, her lung function stabilized, and she found it easier to manage her symptoms. Jane was particularly impressed with how the recipes helped her control inflammation and boost her immune system, allowing her to feel more empowered and confident in managing her condition.

David's Path to Improved Lung Function and Mental Clarity

David, a 57-year-old former smoker, had been battling COPD for several years. His lung capacity had diminished, and he was constantly reliant on inhalers. His physician recommended he make dietary changes, but David had no idea where to start until he came across *The COPD Diet Cookbook*. The nutrient-dense, anti-inflammatory recipes helped him reduce flare-ups and regain control of his breathing. Within a few months, David reported not only improved lung function but also enhanced mental clarity and a newfound sense of well-being. He shared his success story with others, crediting the cookbook with helping him breathe easier and live a more active life.

Lisa's Transformation Through Whole Foods

Lisa, a 45-year-old mother of two, was diagnosed with COPD after years of exposure to environmental pollutants. She had become frustrated with the limitations the disease placed on her life, particularly her ability to keep up with her children. When she started following the meal plans from *The COPD Diet Cookbook*, Lisa saw a dramatic change. The recipes focused on whole foods, lean proteins, and anti-inflammatory ingredients, which helped Lisa feel more in control of her condition. Her lung inflammation decreased, her energy levels soared, and she was able to engage in more physical activities with her family. Lisa's transformation became a testament to the power of nutrition in managing COPD.

Tom's Story of Symptom Management and Weight Control

Tom, a 68-year-old COPD patient, had been dealing with constant shortness of breath and weight gain due to reduced physical activity. The combination of medications and an unhealthy diet was exacerbating his symptoms. After adopting the principles in *The COPD Diet Cookbook*, Tom started seeing improvements. The low-sodium, nutrient-rich recipes helped him control his weight, reduce bloating, and improve his lung function. He particularly appreciated the section on energy-boosting foods that made him feel less fatigued. Over time, Tom was able to walk longer distances, manage his symptoms more effectively, and feel more optimistic about his health.

Chapter 1:

The Fundamentals of a COPD-Friendly Diet

Key Nutrients that Support Lung Health and Boost Energy

To support lung health and energy levels in people with COPD, it's essential to focus on nutrients like antioxidants, vitamins, and minerals. Vitamin C and E, along with selenium and beta-carotene, help combat oxidative stress, which can worsen lung function. Omega-3 fatty acids found in fish like salmon and flaxseeds reduce inflammation, while magnesium-rich foods like spinach improve lung capacity by relaxing the muscles in the airways. Consuming protein from lean meats and legumes provides energy while supporting tissue repair.

To implement these, include colorful fruits like oranges and berries for a daily antioxidant boost, and opt for fatty fish or flaxseed oil for omega-3s. Incorporating leafy greens such as spinach or kale into salads and smoothies ensures a steady intake of magnesium. Regularly consuming these nutrients will promote better lung function and boost energy naturally, supporting overall well-being.

Foods to Include and Avoid for Managing COPD Symptoms

Managing COPD symptoms involves selecting foods that reduce inflammation and support lung function. Focus on including fruits, vegetables, whole grains, and lean proteins. Anti-inflammatory foods like berries, leafy greens, and fatty fish help reduce airway irritation. High-fiber foods such as oats and brown rice aid in digestion, reducing bloating, which can pressure the diaphragm. Avoid processed foods, excessive salt, and refined sugars, as they can contribute to inflammation, water retention, and fatigue.

Practically, this means creating meals with whole ingredients, like a grilled salmon salad with mixed greens and olive oil dressing, while avoiding fast food or processed snacks. Limiting sodium by seasoning with herbs instead of salt can prevent fluid retention, reducing the risk of shortness of breath. These dietary adjustments can significantly improve daily respiratory comfort.

How to Balance Macronutrients for Better Respiratory Function

Balancing macronutrients—proteins, fats, and carbohydrates—can improve breathing in people with COPD. Consuming moderate protein, such as lean chicken, fish, or plant-based proteins like lentils, supports muscle strength, including the respiratory muscles. Carbohydrates, especially complex carbs like whole grains, provide sustained energy, but overconsumption of simple carbs can increase carbon dioxide production, making breathing harder. Healthy fats, such as those from avocados, nuts, and olive oil, are a good energy source without increasing CO_2 levels.

A practical approach is to aim for meals like quinoa bowls with grilled chicken, avocado slices, and roasted vegetables. Limit bread, pasta, or sweets that contain refined carbs, and substitute them with options like brown rice or sweet potatoes. This balance of macronutrients will provide energy without overburdening the lungs, making breathing more efficient.

The Importance of Hydration and How It Affects the Lungs

Staying hydrated is crucial for lung health, especially for those with COPD. Adequate water intake helps thin mucus, making it easier to clear from the lungs and reducing the risk of infections. Dehydration can thicken mucus, making breathing difficult and increasing irritation in the airways. The general recommendation is to drink about 8 cups of water daily, though this may vary based on individual needs.

For practical hydration, carry a water bottle throughout the day and aim to drink small amounts regularly rather than large quantities at once. Herbal teas, low-sodium broths, and water-rich fruits like cucumbers and melons can also contribute to hydration. Avoid caffeinated or sugary drinks, which can dehydrate the body, making it harder to manage COPD symptoms.

Daily Meal Planning Tips to Reduce Inflammation and Mucus Production

Reducing inflammation and mucus production through meal planning involves focusing on whole, unprocessed foods. Start by incorporating anti-inflammatory ingredients like turmeric, ginger, and garlic into dishes. For breakfast, opt for oatmeal with fresh berries and a sprinkle of flaxseed, which is high in omega-3s. Lunch could be a vegetable stir-fry with quinoa, and dinner might include grilled fish with steamed broccoli and sweet potatoes.

To avoid foods that increase mucus, limit dairy products like cheese and milk, as well as processed meats and fried foods. Planning meals helps ensure that you have nutrient-dense, anti-inflammatory foods on hand, reducing the likelihood of resorting to less healthy options. This approach supports lung health and keeps mucus production under control.

Chapter 2:

Best Grocery Store Foods for a COPD Diet

Nutrient-Rich Fruits and Vegetables to Stockpile

To manage COPD, prioritize nutrient-rich fruits and vegetables that support lung health and reduce inflammation. Stockpile dark leafy greens like spinach and kale, which are packed with antioxidants, vitamins A and C, and fiber, all essential for maintaining strong immune function. Add bell peppers, tomatoes, and carrots to your diet for their high vitamin C content, which helps fight respiratory infections. Berries, especially blueberries and strawberries, are excellent sources of antioxidants that protect against oxidative stress in the lungs.

For practical use, incorporate these fruits and vegetables into daily meals. Blend spinach and berries into smoothies, toss leafy greens into salads, or roast carrots and bell peppers as a side dish. For snacks, enjoy raw carrots with a healthy dip or a handful of berries. Keeping these foods readily available will make it easier to include them in your COPD-friendly meal plan.

Whole Grains and Lean Proteins that Support Lung Function

Whole grains like oats, quinoa, and brown rice are high in fiber and provide steady energy without causing blood sugar spikes, which is essential for maintaining stamina when managing COPD. These grains also contain essential nutrients like magnesium and selenium, which aid in respiratory function. Lean proteins, such as chicken, turkey, fish, and plant-based options like beans and tofu, are key for maintaining muscle mass, particularly as COPD can lead to muscle weakness over time.

Incorporate whole grains and lean proteins into your daily meals. Start your day with oatmeal topped with fresh fruit, prepare quinoa or brown rice as a side for lunch or dinner, and pair it with a source of lean protein like grilled chicken or baked fish. For plant-based options, consider a quinoa salad with chickpeas or a tofu stir-fry with vegetables for a balanced meal that promotes lung health.

Healthy Fats that Combat Inflammation and Enhance Energy

Healthy fats, particularly omega-3 fatty acids, are essential for reducing inflammation in the lungs and providing long-lasting energy. Incorporate fatty fish like salmon, mackerel, and sardines into your diet, as they are rich in omega-3s. Other great sources include flaxseeds, chia seeds, walnuts, and olive oil. These fats not only combat inflammation but also help maintain energy levels, which is crucial for managing COPD symptoms like fatigue.

To add healthy fats to your meals, drizzle olive oil over salads or roasted vegetables, and sprinkle chia or flaxseeds into smoothies or yogurt. Snack on a handful of walnuts or make a quick tuna salad with olive oil and lemon. By incorporating these healthy fats daily, you'll improve lung function and boost overall energy levels without resorting to processed, inflammatory fats.

How to Read Food Labels and Choose COPD-Friendly Products

When managing COPD, reading food labels is key to avoiding ingredients that may trigger inflammation or worsen symptoms. Focus on sodium content, as excessive salt can lead to fluid retention and make breathing difficult. Aim for products with less than 140 mg of sodium per serving. Avoid processed foods with added sugars, which can increase inflammation and contribute to weight gain. Instead, opt for whole foods with minimal ingredients, such as fresh vegetables, whole grains, and lean proteins.

To choose COPD-friendly products, look for items labeled as "low-sodium," "low-sugar," or "whole grain." Check ingredient lists for added preservatives, artificial colors, and unhealthy fats, which can increase inflammation. For example, when buying canned vegetables, choose "no salt added" varieties, and for bread or cereal, opt for whole grain options without added sugars. Reading labels carefully ensures you're making choices that support your lung health.

Tips for Organizing a COPD-Friendly Pantry

A well-organized pantry can make it easier to stick to a COPD-friendly diet. Start by clearing out foods high in sodium, sugar, and unhealthy fats, such as processed snacks, sugary cereals, and canned goods with added salt. Replace them with COPD-friendly staples like whole grains (quinoa, brown rice, oats), low-sodium canned vegetables, lean protein sources (canned tuna, beans), and healthy fats (olive oil, nuts). Organize these items in easy-to-reach areas to encourage healthy meal prep.

Group similar items together for convenience. For example, store all your whole grains in one section and your protein sources in another. Use clear containers to keep snacks like nuts and seeds visible and accessible. Label shelves or containers to quickly find what you need. By keeping your pantry stocked and organized with COPD-friendly foods, you'll simplify meal planning and reduce the temptation to reach for less healthy options.

Chapter 3:

Appetizers for Lung Health

Easy-to-Digest Starters That Promote Better Breathing

To improve breathing and manage COPD, it's important to start meals with foods that are easy to digest and gentle on the lungs. Opt for dishes like blended vegetable soups or mashed sweet potatoes, which are nutrient-rich yet easy to break down, minimizing bloating and discomfort. Avoid heavy creams or fried options, and instead, use olive oil or broth-based starters that can help with inflammation and promote smooth digestion.

One easy recipe could be a carrot and ginger soup, lightly seasoned with herbs and blended to a smooth consistency. Carrots are packed with beta-carotene, which supports lung function, while ginger has anti-inflammatory properties that help with breathing. Simply sauté carrots and ginger in olive oil, add vegetable broth, and blend until smooth. This starter provides a light, lung-friendly option to kick off a meal.

Incorporating Herbs and Spices That Fight Inflammation

Herbs and spices such as turmeric, garlic, and rosemary are potent anti-inflammatory agents that can benefit those with COPD by reducing airway inflammation. Adding these into meals not only enhances flavor but also helps manage symptoms. For example, turmeric can be mixed into soups, and stews, or sprinkled on roasted vegetables, while garlic can be sautéed in olive oil to serve as the base for many dishes.

A simple dish like roasted cauliflower with turmeric and black pepper combines flavor and health benefits. Turmeric's active compound, curcumin, is known for its anti-inflammatory properties, and black pepper enhances its absorption. This makes it an easy way to incorporate medicinal spices into daily meals while managing COPD symptoms.

Low-Sodium Appetizer Options for COPD Management

For people managing COPD, reducing sodium intake is crucial to prevent fluid retention, which can worsen breathing. Opt for appetizers that use natural herbs and spices instead of salt for flavor. Try a simple cucumber and dill salad, using Greek yogurt for creaminess instead of salty dressings. Cucumber helps hydrate the body, and dill adds flavor without the need for salt.

Another quick option is roasted chickpeas seasoned with smoked paprika and garlic powder. Chickpeas provide fiber and protein, while spices offer bold flavors without added sodium. These low-sodium, easy-to-make appetizers help manage COPD without sacrificing taste.

Nutrient-dense, Light Appetizers for Easy Digestion

To ensure easy digestion while providing essential nutrients, choose light, nutrient-dense appetizers such as avocado-based dishes or spinach and fruit salads. Avocado is rich in healthy fats that support energy and lung health, while spinach offers a good dose of vitamins like A and C, which are essential for respiratory wellness. Combine avocado slices with a drizzle of lemon juice and fresh herbs for a refreshing starter.

A spinach and strawberry salad with a light vinaigrette dressing can also be a great option. Spinach offers iron and antioxidants, while strawberries provide vitamin C, which boosts immune function and supports lung health. Both options are light on the stomach, making them easy to digest while still packing a nutritional punch.

Quick and Simple Recipes to Prepare on Busy Days

On busy days, it's essential to have quick and simple recipes that don't compromise on nutrition. An example is an avocado toast topped with a boiled egg and a sprinkle of pepper. It's quick to prepare, nutrient-dense, and easy to digest, making it an ideal meal for those managing COPD. The healthy fats from the avocado and the protein from the egg provide energy without the heaviness that might affect breathing.

Another quick option is a quinoa salad mixed with chopped veggies and a drizzle of olive oil and lemon juice. Quinoa cooks in about 15 minutes and is high in protein and fiber, which helps keep you full without feeling bloated. The combination of nutrient-rich vegetables and whole grains supports lung function and provides energy for the day.

Chapter 4:

Energizing Breakfast Recipes for COPD

Breakfast Foods That Provide Lasting Energy throughout the Day

For a breakfast that sustains energy, opt for whole grains, proteins, and healthy fats. Start your day with oatmeal topped with nuts and seeds, which provides slow-digesting carbohydrates for steady energy. Whole grain toast with avocado and a poached egg is another excellent choice, combining complex carbs and healthy fats. These options release energy gradually, preventing the mid-morning slump often caused by sugary foods.

Another effective way to maintain energy is incorporating high-protein foods like Greek yogurt with berries and a sprinkle of chia seeds. This combination provides a balance of protein, fiber, and antioxidants, supporting both your energy levels and overall lung health. Balancing your meals with the right nutrients is key to keeping your energy up throughout the day.

Low-Sugar, High-Fiber Options to Support Lung Health

To support lung health, choose breakfast options low in sugar but rich in fiber, such as a bowl of quinoa porridge with fresh berries and a handful of almonds. This meal is high in fiber and antioxidants, helping to reduce inflammation and improve digestion without spiking blood sugar levels. Avoid sugary cereals and opt for whole grains that offer long-lasting energy while supporting healthy lung function.

Another option is a slice of whole-grain bread topped with hummus and cucumber slices, paired with a small apple. The fiber content of both the bread and apple helps maintain blood sugar levels while promoting lung health. Additionally, fiber-rich foods improve digestion, which indirectly supports respiratory wellness.

Quick Breakfast Smoothies Packed with Essential Nutrients

For a nutrient-packed breakfast on the go, blend a smoothie with leafy greens like spinach or kale, half a banana, and a handful of frozen berries. Add a scoop of plant-based protein powder and a tablespoon of flaxseeds or chia seeds for extra fiber and omega-3s. This combination delivers vitamins, minerals, and antioxidants that help fight inflammation and support lung function.

To make it even more balanced, you can also add almond milk or a bit of yogurt to provide healthy fats and probiotics for better digestion. Smoothies are an excellent way to quickly intake nutrients, and they are easy to customize based on your taste preferences and nutritional needs.

Incorporating Healthy Fats for a Satisfying Morning Meal

Incorporating healthy fats into your breakfast can help you stay full and energized longer. Start with a bowl of plain Greek yogurt mixed with flaxseeds and topped with avocado slices. The combination of monounsaturated fats from the avocado and omega-3s from flaxseeds supports heart and lung health while providing lasting satiety.

Alternatively, you can try scrambled eggs cooked in olive oil, served with a slice of smoked salmon and avocado on whole-grain toast. The healthy fats from olive oil and avocado combined with the protein in eggs and salmon create a balanced and satisfying meal, perfect for maintaining energy and lung function throughout the day.

Anti-Inflammatory Ingredients to Kick-Start the Day

Anti-inflammatory foods can be easily integrated into breakfast to improve lung health. Try making a warm turmeric oatmeal by adding a pinch of turmeric, cinnamon, and ginger to your oats. These spices are known for their anti-inflammatory properties, which can help reduce lung irritation and improve breathing over time.

You can also create an anti-inflammatory smoothie by blending frozen blueberries, spinach, a teaspoon of turmeric, and almond milk. Blueberries and spinach are rich in antioxidants that protect against inflammation, while turmeric adds an extra boost of respiratory support. These breakfasts are quick, flavorful, and packed with ingredients that promote overall wellness.

Chapter 5:

Lung-Friendly Smoothie Recipes

Best Fruits and Vegetables to Include in COPD-Friendly Smoothies

For COPD-friendly smoothies, it's important to focus on fruits and vegetables that are high in antioxidants, vitamins, and minerals that support lung health. Some of the best fruits to include are berries like strawberries, blueberries, and raspberries, which are rich in vitamin C and antioxidants that help reduce inflammation in the lungs. Bananas provide potassium, aiding in electrolyte balance, while oranges are packed with vitamin C to support the immune system. Vegetables like spinach, kale, and carrots are also excellent because they provide fiber, vitamin A, and other essential nutrients that contribute to respiratory wellness.

To prepare, simply blend a mix of these fruits and vegetables with a base like almond milk or water. For example, a smoothie with spinach, banana, and berries creates a nutrient-rich, COPD-friendly drink. Adding leafy greens like kale provides antioxidants, while carrots contribute beta-carotene, which converts to vitamin A, crucial for lung tissue repair.

Adding Protein to Smoothies for Energy and Muscle Strength

Protein is essential for people with COPD as it helps maintain muscle mass, which can decline with the condition. Adding a scoop of protein powder, such as whey, pea, or hemp protein, to your smoothie is an easy way to boost energy and support muscle strength. Yogurt and nut butter, like almond or peanut butter, are also excellent sources of protein that blend smoothly into shakes. Greek yogurt, in particular, adds both protein and probiotics, which help improve gut health.

You can also incorporate plant-based protein sources like chia seeds, flaxseeds, or silken tofu. For instance, a smoothie with banana, spinach, almond butter, and a scoop of whey protein provides a balanced blend of macronutrients. This combination delivers not only protein but also fiber and healthy fats, keeping you full and energized throughout the day.

How to Make Smoothies That Are Easy to Digest and Reduce Inflammation

To make smoothies that are easy to digest and reduce inflammation, it's important to select ingredients that are gentle on the stomach and have anti-inflammatory properties. Start with fruits like papaya and pineapple, which contain digestive enzymes that aid indigestion. Ginger is another excellent addition due to its anti-inflammatory and soothing properties. Use a liquid base like coconut water or almond milk, which are lighter and easier to digest compared to dairy.

Additionally, avoid adding too many fibrous vegetables that might cause bloating, such as raw kale or broccoli. Instead, choose cooked or steamed vegetables like zucchini or carrots, which are gentler on the digestive system. A great example of an anti-inflammatory smoothie is blending pineapple, ginger, and spinach with coconut water. This creates a refreshing, easy-to-digest drink that also helps to reduce lung inflammation.

Smoothie Recipes Tailored to Boost Respiratory Function

Creating smoothies to enhance respiratory function involves selecting ingredients that support lung health. A good combination would include fruits and vegetables rich in antioxidants, like berries, spinach, and citrus fruits. For example, a blend of blueberries, spinach, and orange juice creates a smoothie that is packed with vitamins C and E, both of which are crucial for protecting lung tissue from damage and improving overall lung function.

Another example is combining banana, kale, and ginger for a smoothie that delivers potassium, fiber, and anti-inflammatory benefits, all of which support better breathing. For extra respiratory support, add a teaspoon of turmeric, which is known for its powerful anti-inflammatory effects, helping to soothe airways and reduce symptoms of COPD.

Tips for Preparing Smoothies in Advance for Convenience

To make smoothie preparation easier, you can prepare the ingredients in advance and store them for quick use. One method is to pre-portion your fruits, vegetables, and other add-ins like protein powder or seeds into freezer bags. Label the bags with the recipe and just grab a bag, add liquid, and blend when needed. This makes it incredibly convenient, especially on busy days when you want a healthy option but don't have time to prepare everything from scratch.

Another tip is to blend a large batch of smoothies and store them in mason jars or airtight containers in the fridge. Smoothies can generally last 1-2 days when stored this way. To keep them fresh, you can add a squeeze of lemon juice, which slows down oxidation. Just give the jar a good shake before drinking, and your smoothie will be ready to go!

Chapter 6:

Lunch Recipes to Boost Lung Function

Easy-to-Make Lunches with Nutrient-Dense Ingredients

Creating nutrient-dense lunches doesn't need to be complicated. A simple quinoa salad with avocado, spinach, and grilled chicken packs essential vitamins, minerals, and healthy fats, all vital for lung health. Combine a handful of fresh vegetables, lean protein, and a splash of olive oil for a quick, wholesome meal. Another easy option is a turkey and hummus wrap with whole-grain tortilla, providing a good balance of protein, fiber, and healthy fats.

Smoothie bowls can also be a fast lunch option, blending spinach, banana, almond butter, and chia seeds for a nutrient-packed meal. Top with flaxseeds and berries to boost the fiber and antioxidant content, which supports respiratory function. These recipes are quick to prepare and deliver the nutrients needed for managing COPD while maintaining energy levels throughout the day.

Lean Protein Options that Support Muscle Strength

For maintaining muscle strength and supporting respiratory health, lean proteins like chicken breast, turkey, and fish are excellent choices. A grilled chicken breast served over a bed of greens with a drizzle of balsamic vinaigrette offers a simple, protein-rich lunch. Add some quinoa or barley to boost the fiber content, which aids digestion and sustains energy levels.

Eggs are another fantastic, lean protein source. Try making a veggie-filled omelet with spinach, tomatoes, and mushrooms, or hard-boiled eggs as a grab-and-go option. Beans and lentils can also be incorporated into soups or salads for plant-based protein, promoting muscle health while aiding in managing COPD symptoms.

Whole Grain and Fiber-Rich Recipes for Optimal Digestion

Whole grains like brown rice, quinoa, and barley are fiber-rich options that support digestion and help stabilize blood sugar levels, which is essential for COPD management. A brown rice and black bean bowl topped with salsa, avocado, and a sprinkle of cheese offers a high-fiber, nutrient-packed meal that's quick and filling.

Oat-based dishes are also great for lunches. A savory oatmeal with spinach, a soft-boiled egg, and a sprinkle of seeds provides a fiber boost while keeping energy levels steady. The fiber in whole grains helps manage cholesterol levels, reduces inflammation, and supports overall respiratory health.

Anti-Inflammatory Lunch Ideas for Managing COPD Symptoms

Managing inflammation is crucial for COPD, and certain foods can help. A salmon salad with spinach, avocado, and a sprinkle of walnuts offers anti-inflammatory omega-3s, fiber, and antioxidants that aid in reducing lung inflammation. You can prepare this quickly by using canned wild salmon, tossed with leafy greens and olive oil.

Chickpeas and turmeric soup is another anti-inflammatory option. Turmeric, known for its curcumin content, helps fight inflammation, while chickpeas provide a good source of protein and fiber. Simply simmer chickpeas with vegetable broth, turmeric, garlic, and ginger for a flavorful, health-boosting lunch that's gentle on the lungs.

Simple Lunch Options that Keep Energy Levels Stable

Maintaining steady energy throughout the day is crucial, especially for those with COPD. A whole-grain wrap filled with lean turkey, hummus, and fresh veggies like cucumber and lettuce offers a balanced meal rich in fiber, protein, and healthy fats, ensuring a slow release of energy without blood sugar spikes.

Greek yogurt with mixed nuts, berries, and a drizzle of honey is another easy, energy-boosting option. It provides a good balance of protein, healthy fats, and natural sugars to keep you full and energized. Both these options are quick to assemble, making them perfect for busy days when you need a nutritious lunch to fuel your afternoon.

Chapter 7:

Snacking Strategies for COPD

Healthy Snack Options That Won't Leave You Breathless

For individuals with COPD, choosing snacks that are easy to digest and won't exacerbate symptoms is crucial. Opt for snacks that are light and low in added sugars and fats, such as fresh fruits like apples or pears, and vegetables like carrot sticks or cucumber slices. These options provide essential vitamins and minerals without causing discomfort or breathlessness.

In addition, consider snacks with anti-inflammatory properties, such as berries and leafy greens. These foods can help reduce inflammation in the respiratory system and are generally easier on the lungs, ensuring you stay comfortable while snacking.

High-Protein, Low-Sodium Snacks for Sustained Energy

High-protein snacks are essential for maintaining energy levels and muscle mass, particularly for those with COPD. Choose lean proteins like turkey slices, low-fat Greek yogurt, or cottage cheese. These options offer sustained energy without the high sodium content that can lead to fluid retention and worsen COPD symptoms.

Incorporate plant-based proteins as well, such as hummus or edamame. These snacks are not only protein-rich but also low in sodium, making them an excellent choice for keeping energy levels stable while managing symptoms effectively.

Incorporating Nuts and Seeds to Boost Nutrition

Nuts and seeds are packed with healthy fats, fiber, and essential nutrients that can support lung health. Almonds, walnuts, chia seeds, and flaxseeds are particularly beneficial. They provide omega-3 fatty acids, which have anti-inflammatory properties and can improve respiratory function.

To enjoy nuts and seeds, consider adding them to yogurt, salads, or as a topping for whole-grain toast. They can also be blended into smoothies for an extra boost of nutrition without overwhelming the digestive system.

How to Prepare Grab-and-Go Snacks for Busy Days

For busy days, preparation is key. Create snack packs in advance by portioning out snacks like sliced veggies, fruit, or mixed nuts into small containers. This ensures you have quick, healthy options readily available without needing to prepare something on the spot.

Use resealable bags or containers to keep snacks fresh and portable. Consider making a large batch of these snacks at the beginning of the week to save time and ensure you always have COPD-friendly options on hand.

COPD-Friendly Snack Recipes to Manage Cravings

To manage cravings while adhering to a COPD-friendly diet, try recipes that are easy to prepare and align with dietary needs. For instance, a blend of low-fat Greek yogurt with fresh fruit and a sprinkle of nuts can be both satisfying and beneficial.

Another option is to make a batch of homemade energy balls using oats, nut butter, and a touch of honey. These provide a quick, nutritious snack that supports energy levels and lung health while helping to curb unhealthy cravings.

Chapter 8:

Dinner Recipes for Respiratory Wellness

Balanced Dinners that Support Lung Function and Overall Health

When preparing balanced dinners for optimal lung health, focus on incorporating a variety of nutrients that support respiratory function. Include plenty of fruits, vegetables, whole grains, and lean proteins. For instance, a meal could consist of baked salmon, quinoa, and a side of steamed broccoli. The salmon provides omega-3 fatty acids, which help reduce inflammation, while the quinoa and broccoli contribute essential vitamins and minerals for overall health.

Another effective strategy is to use healthy fats like olive oil and avocado in your cooking. These fats support cellular health and can aid in reducing inflammation. An example would be a mixed greens salad with avocado slices and a drizzle of olive oil, paired with a grilled chicken breast. This combination ensures you get a balance of healthy fats, lean protein, and a variety of nutrients to support lung function.

Low-Carb, High-Fiber Dinner Options to Reduce Inflammation

Opting for low-carb, high-fiber dinners can help manage inflammation associated with COPD. Vegetables like spinach, kale, and cauliflower are excellent choices due to their high fiber content and low carbohydrate levels. A great meal idea is a cauliflower rice stir-fry with mixed vegetables and a small portion of tofu or chicken. This meal is low in carbs, high in fiber, and provides a good dose of antioxidants.

Incorporating legumes such as lentils and chickpeas into your meals can also be beneficial. These foods are high in fiber and protein while being low in carbs. A simple dish might include a lentil and vegetable stew. This meal not only helps in reducing inflammation but also keeps you full and satisfied due to its high fiber content.

Lean Protein Sources that Help Maintain Muscle Mass

Maintaining muscle mass is crucial for people with COPD, and lean protein sources are essential for this purpose. Foods like chicken breast, turkey, fish, and legumes are excellent options. For example, a dinner of grilled chicken breast served with a side of steamed asparagus and a small portion of brown rice provides lean protein and essential nutrients that support muscle maintenance. Another good source of lean protein is beans and lentils, which can be used in various dishes. A tasty and nutritious option is a chickpea and spinach curry. This dish offers high protein content from the chickpeas and additional nutrients from the spinach, supporting muscle health and overall vitality.

Tips for Incorporating COPD-Friendly Spices and Herbs into Meals

Spices and herbs can enhance the flavor of your meals without adding extra salt or fat, which is beneficial for COPD patients. Opt for herbs like basil, thyme, and rosemary, which add a burst of flavor and provide anti-inflammatory benefits. For instance, seasoning a roasted vegetable dish with rosemary and thyme can make it more flavorful while supporting lung health.

Turmeric and ginger are also excellent choices due to their anti-inflammatory properties. Incorporate them into your cooking by adding a pinch of turmeric to soups or using ginger in stir-fries. These spices not only enhance taste but also contribute to reducing inflammation and improving respiratory wellness.

Easy-to-Make, Delicious Recipes for Satisfying Dinners

Creating easy and satisfying dinners is achievable with simple recipes that focus on wholesome ingredients. Try a recipe for a quinoa and vegetable stuffed bell pepper. To make it, cook quinoa, mix it with diced vegetables like tomatoes and onions, stuff the mixture into bell peppers, and bake until tender. This dish is nutritious, easy to prepare, and delicious.

Another quick and healthy option is a salmon and avocado wrap. Simply grill a salmon fillet, slice it, and wrap it in a whole-grain tortilla with avocado slices and a handful of spinach. This meal is not only straightforward to make but also packed with nutrients that support lung health and overall well-being.

Chapter 9:

Desserts that Support Lung Health

Low-Sugar Dessert Options That Won't Aggravate Symptoms

When managing COPD, choosing desserts with low sugar content can help prevent exacerbation of symptoms. Opt for desserts made with natural sweeteners like stevia or monk fruit instead of refined sugars. For example, try a chia seed pudding sweetened with a small amount of honey or maple syrup. The chia seeds provide fiber and omega-3 fatty acids, which support overall lung health.

Another option is baked goods using whole grains and reduced sugar. Consider making oatmeal cookies with unsweetened applesauce as a sugar substitute. This method reduces the sugar content while adding fiber, which is beneficial for digestion and energy levels. Always read labels carefully to ensure that no hidden sugars or unhealthy additives are included.

Anti-Inflammatory Dessert Recipes with COPD-Friendly Ingredients

Incorporating anti-inflammatory ingredients into desserts can help manage COPD symptoms. Use ingredients like turmeric, ginger, and berries, which have anti-inflammatory properties. For instance, a berry smoothie with spinach and a pinch of turmeric provides a refreshing treat while reducing inflammation.

Try making a homemade apple crisp using cinnamon and ginger. These spices have natural anti-inflammatory benefits and can be paired with a whole-grain or nut-based crumble topping to enhance the nutritional value. Avoid processed ingredients and opt for whole, fresh foods to maximize the anti-inflammatory benefits.

Incorporating Fruit and Healthy Fats into Sweet Treats

Fruits and healthy fats can add flavor and nutrition to COPD-friendly desserts. Incorporate fruits like berries, apples, and bananas into recipes for added vitamins and antioxidants. For example, make a banana and berry frozen yogurt by blending frozen fruit with Greek yogurt and a touch of vanilla extract.

Include healthy fats like avocados and nuts to enhance the nutritional profile of desserts. An avocado-based chocolate mousse, made with cocoa powder and a natural sweetener, provides a creamy, satisfying dessert rich in healthy fats and antioxidants. This combination helps maintain energy levels and supports overall lung function.

Simple Dessert Ideas to Satisfy Cravings Without Overindulging

Simple and healthy desserts can help satisfy cravings without compromising COPD management. Prepare a fruit salad with a variety of fresh, seasonal fruits, and a squeeze of lemon juice for added flavor without extra calories. This option is quick to make and provides natural sweetness and essential nutrients.

Another easy dessert is a yogurt parfait layered with fresh fruit and a sprinkle of nuts or seeds. Greek yogurt offers protein and probiotics, while the fruit adds vitamins and fiber. This combination makes for a filling and nutritious treat that won't lead to overindulgence.

How to Enjoy Dessert While Managing COPD Effectively

To enjoy desserts while managing COPD, focus on portion control and ingredient choices. Opt for small servings of nutrient-dense desserts to avoid overconsumption of calories and sugars. For example, a small serving of almond flour cake can satisfy a sweet tooth without overwhelming the digestive system.

Additionally, choose desserts that align with your overall dietary goals. Select recipes that use ingredients beneficial for lung health, such as fruits, vegetables, and whole grains. Balance these treats with a well-rounded diet and monitor your body's response to ensure that your choices support your COPD management effectively.

Chapter 10:

Vegetarian Recipes for COPD

Plant-Based Protein Sources That Boost Lung Health

Incorporating plant-based protein sources into your diet can significantly support lung health. Beans, lentils, quinoa, and tofu are excellent options that provide essential amino acids without the saturated fats found in animal products. For instance, a hearty lentil soup or a quinoa and black bean salad can be both nutritious and beneficial for your respiratory system. These proteins help repair lung tissues and support overall immune function, which is crucial for managing COPD.

Additionally, nuts and seeds, such as chia seeds and almonds, offer a protein boost and are packed with healthy fats that help reduce inflammation in the body. Adding a handful of almonds to your breakfast oatmeal or sprinkling chia seeds on a smoothie can enhance your intake of these lung-supportive nutrients.

High-Fiber Vegetarian Meals to Support Digestion and Energy Levels

High-fiber meals are essential for maintaining digestive health and boosting energy levels, which is especially important for those with COPD. Foods like whole grains, vegetables, fruits, and legumes are rich in fiber. A whole-grain vegetable stir-fry or a mixed bean chili can keep your digestive system functioning smoothly and provide sustained energy throughout the day.

For added fiber, consider including foods such as avocados and sweet potatoes in your diet. These ingredients not only promote good digestion but also help stabilize blood sugar levels, which can enhance overall energy and prevent fatigue.

How to Balance Carbohydrates and Protein in Vegetarian Dishes

Balancing carbohydrates and protein in vegetarian dishes ensures that you get a well-rounded meal that supports lung health and overall energy. Aim for a ratio where half your plate is filled with vegetables, a quarter with protein sources like beans or tofu, and a quarter with whole grains such as brown rice or quinoa. This combination helps maintain steady energy levels and prevents blood sugar spikes.

For example, a dish like a quinoa and chickpea salad combines protein-rich quinoa and chickpeas with fiber-packed vegetables, ensuring a balanced intake of both macronutrients. Adjusting portion sizes based on your personal energy needs can also help in maintaining this balance.

Anti-Inflammatory Vegetarian Ingredients to Incorporate Into Meals

Including anti-inflammatory ingredients in your meals can be beneficial for managing COPD symptoms. Foods such as turmeric, ginger, and leafy greens like spinach and kale have been shown to reduce inflammation. Adding turmeric to a vegetable curry or incorporating ginger into a smoothie can provide these anti-inflammatory benefits.

Additionally, berries, such as blueberries and strawberries, are high in antioxidants and can help combat oxidative stress. You might enjoy a mixed berry smoothie or add berries to your breakfast yogurt for a flavorful and health-boosting start to the day.

Easy-to-Make, Lung-Friendly Vegetarian Recipes

Preparing lung-friendly vegetarian meals doesn't have to be complicated. Simple recipes such as a roasted vegetable medley with quinoa or lentil and spinach stew are not only nutritious but also easy to make. These recipes often require just a few ingredients and basic cooking techniques, making them ideal for busy individuals looking to improve their lung health.

Chapter 11:

Hydration and Its Impact on COPD

The Importance of Proper Hydration for Lung Health

Hydration plays a crucial role in maintaining lung health by ensuring that mucus in the airways remains thin and easier to expel. Proper hydration helps keep the mucous membranes in the lungs moist, which can aid in preventing infections and reducing inflammation. For those with COPD, keeping mucus thin is particularly important to avoid coughing and difficulty breathing.

Drinking enough fluids also helps to maintain overall bodily functions, including the respiratory system. It supports the efficient delivery of oxygen to cells and helps in the removal of waste products. Ensuring proper hydration can significantly improve comfort and respiratory function in individuals with COPD.

Best Beverages to Include in a COPD-Friendly Diet

In a COPD-friendly diet, aim to include beverages that are low in sugar and high in nutrients. Water is the best choice, as it hydrates without adding calories or sugar. Herbal teas, such as ginger or peppermint, can also be beneficial due to their anti-inflammatory properties. Additionally, low-sodium broths can help with hydration while also providing essential minerals.

Avoid caffeinated and alcoholic beverages as they can lead to dehydration. Opt for beverages that offer added health benefits, such as green tea, which has antioxidants that may support lung health. Smoothies made with nutrient-rich ingredients can also be a great choice for hydration and overall well-being.

How Dehydration Can Worsen COPD Symptoms

Dehydration can exacerbate COPD symptoms by thickening mucus, making it harder to clear from the airways. This can lead to increased coughing, wheezing, and difficulty breathing. When mucus becomes thick and sticky, it can cause blockages in the airways, worsening respiratory issues and leading to potential infections.

Additionally, dehydration can impact overall health, leading to fatigue and decreased energy levels, which can affect the ability to manage COPD symptoms effectively. Staying well-hydrated helps in maintaining a more comfortable and manageable respiratory condition.

Tips for Increasing Fluid Intake Throughout the Day

To increase fluid intake, set regular reminders to drink water throughout the day. Carry a reusable water bottle with you to ensure easy access to fluids and track your intake. Incorporate water-rich foods into your diet, such as fruits and vegetables, which can contribute to your overall hydration.

Consider setting daily hydration goals and using apps or journals to monitor your progress. Drinking smaller amounts frequently rather than large amounts at once can be more effective and less overwhelming, helping to maintain steady hydration levels throughout the day.

Hydrating Smoothie and Soup Recipes for Respiratory Wellness

Smoothies can be a fantastic way to boost hydration while providing essential nutrients. Try blending spinach, cucumber, and a splash of lemon juice for a refreshing, hydrating drink. Add a handful of berries for added antioxidants and vitamins that support lung health.

For soups, consider recipes like a clear vegetable broth with carrots, celery, and spinach. These soups not only hydrate but also provide vitamins and minerals that are beneficial for respiratory wellness. Avoid adding excess salt to keep the broth healthy and supportive of lung function.

Chapter 12:

Anti-Inflammatory Spices and Herbs for COPD

Best Anti-Inflammatory Herbs and Spices to Use in Cooking

Anti-inflammatory herbs and spices like turmeric, ginger, garlic, and cinnamon are powerful additions to a COPD-friendly diet. Turmeric, with its active compound curcumin, has been shown to reduce lung inflammation, making it a great option for soups, stews, or sprinkled over roasted vegetables. Ginger and garlic also possess anti-inflammatory properties, making them ideal for enhancing the flavors of stir-fries, marinades, and salad dressings.

To make the most of these spices, use them fresh or ground in everyday cooking. For example, adding freshly grated ginger to smoothies or using garlic in homemade sauces provides not only flavor but also lung-boosting benefits. These herbs are versatile and can be incorporated easily without altering the natural taste of meals. When cooking, remember to pair turmeric with black pepper to enhance curcumin absorption.

How to Incorporate Turmeric, Ginger, and Garlic into Meals

Adding turmeric, ginger, and garlic into daily meals is simple and beneficial for managing COPD symptoms. For breakfast, sprinkle turmeric into scrambled eggs or oatmeal for a golden hue and anti-inflammatory benefits. Add a pinch of ground ginger to smoothies or herbal teas for a zingy flavor that supports lung health. At lunch or dinner, sauté vegetables or chicken with garlic and ginger to infuse your dish with rich, fragrant aromas while promoting respiratory wellness.

For a quick snack, mix turmeric with roasted chickpeas or popcorn for a flavorful, nutrient-rich treat. Garlic can be used in salad dressings or as a base for soups and stews, while ginger works well in marinades or infused in water for a refreshing and healing drink. These ingredients blend seamlessly into various cuisines, from Asian stir-fries to Mediterranean pasta dishes, making it easy to boost your health without overhauling your cooking style.

The Benefits of Antioxidant-Rich Herbs for Lung Health

Antioxidant-rich herbs such as oregano, rosemary, thyme, and basil are potent protectors of lung health. These herbs contain vitamins and phytonutrients that help neutralize free radicals, reduce oxidative stress, and support the immune system. Oregano, for example, contains rosmarinic acid, which helps combat inflammation and infections in the respiratory system. Similarly, thyme has been used for centuries to treat lung conditions due to its antiseptic and anti-inflammatory properties.

Incorporating these herbs into your meals is easy and enhances both flavor and nutrition. Fresh rosemary and thyme can be added to roasted meats, vegetables, or sauces, while oregano and basil work beautifully in salads, soups, or homemade pesto. Regular use of these antioxidant-rich herbs not only enhances the taste of your dishes but also strengthens your lung defenses against environmental toxins.

Recipes That Use Herbs and Spices to Enhance Flavor and Reduce Inflammation

Incorporating anti-inflammatory herbs and spices into recipes can make meals both delicious and beneficial for lung health. For a quick, flavorful dish, try a turmeric and ginger vegetable stir-fry, where you sauté a mix of vegetables in olive oil, garlic, and fresh ginger, finishing with a dash of turmeric. This dish can be paired with brown rice or quinoa for a nutritious meal. Another idea is a garlic and herb-baked salmon, where garlic, rosemary, and thyme are used to season the fish before baking, providing anti-inflammatory and antioxidant benefits in every bite.

Herbs like oregano and basil also work well in homemade soups, such as tomato and basil soup enhanced with fresh oregano and garlic. These recipes offer a great way to reduce inflammation while enjoying comforting, flavorful meals. Pair these meals with whole grains and healthy fats like olive oil to maximize nutrient absorption and support overall wellness.

Herbal Teas That Soothe the Lungs and Improve Breathing

Herbal teas such as peppermint, ginger, and licorice root are excellent for soothing the lungs and promoting easier breathing. Peppermint tea contains menthol, which helps relax the muscles of the respiratory tract, making it easier to breathe, while ginger tea is known for its anti-inflammatory effects and ability to break down mucus in the lungs. Licorice root, often used in traditional medicine, helps to coat and soothe the throat and reduce inflammation in the airways.

To prepare these teas, simply steep fresh or dried herbs in hot water for 5-10 minutes. For added flavor and benefit, mix peppermint with a slice of fresh ginger or combine licorice root with chamomile for a calming evening tea. Drinking these herbal infusions regularly can help reduce lung irritation, clear the airways, and support overall respiratory health.

Chapter 13:

Cooking Techniques to Maximize Nutrition

How to Cook COPD-Friendly Meals Without Losing Nutrients

To cook meals that benefit COPD patients without losing essential nutrients, focus on minimal processing and gentle cooking techniques. Steaming and poaching are excellent options because they prevent vitamin loss compared to frying or boiling, which can leach nutrients into the water or oil. For example, lightly steam vegetables until just tender instead of boiling them, which preserves vitamins like C and B. Use fresh herbs and lemon juice to season, avoiding overcooking, as this depletes key nutrients like antioxidants that support lung health.

Another effective approach is cooking in small batches to avoid reheating, which diminishes nutrients over time. Preparing meals like stir-fries, where ingredients cook quickly at high heat, can maintain more vitamins and minerals than slow cooking. Additionally, adding raw nutrient-dense foods like spinach or bell peppers at the end of cooking helps ensure these ingredients retain their maximum vitamin content.

Best Cooking Methods to Preserve Vitamins and Minerals

Preserving vitamins and minerals while cooking is crucial for COPD patients. Steaming is one of the best methods as it exposes food to minimal heat and water, preventing the breakdown of water-soluble vitamins like vitamin C and folate. For example, using a steam basket for broccoli or carrots helps retain their vibrant color and nutritional value compared to boiling. Another effective technique is sautéing with minimal oil, which maintains nutrients while adding healthy fats that help the body absorb fat-soluble vitamins like A, D, E, and K.

Roasting vegetables and lean proteins at a moderate temperature can also be beneficial. By using parchment paper or aluminum foil, you lock in moisture without needing excess oil. For instance, roasting sweet potatoes or chicken in the oven helps maintain their nutrient density while giving them a rich, caramelized flavor. Avoid deep-frying or cooking at very high temperatures, which can destroy delicate vitamins and increase harmful compounds.

Low-Sodium Cooking Tips for Better Lung Health

For individuals with COPD, reducing sodium is essential to managing symptoms like breathlessness and fluid retention. Use herbs, spices, and natural flavor enhancers like lemon juice, garlic, and ginger to season food without relying on salt. For instance, a sprinkle of fresh thyme or rosemary can add flavor to baked chicken without needing any added sodium. Vinegar, like balsamic or apple cider, also adds depth to dishes while supporting lung health through their antioxidant properties.

Another tip is to rinse canned vegetables, beans, or legumes under water to remove excess sodium. Opting for fresh or frozen produce over canned alternatives helps lower sodium intake, as does choosing unsalted nuts, seeds, and grains. When baking, replace salted butter with unsalted versions and use potassium-rich ingredients like avocados and bananas, which help counteract the effects of sodium on the body.

How to Prepare Meals That Are Easy to Chew and Digest

For COPD patients who may have difficulty chewing or digesting food, preparing soft, easily manageable meals is crucial. Use slow-cooking methods like braising or stewing to make lean meats and vegetables tender. For example, preparing a chicken and vegetable stew allows the ingredients to soften without losing their nutritional value. Blending or mashing foods, such as making mashed sweet potatoes or smoothies with spinach and bananas, also offers nutritious and easy-to-consume options.

Another approach is to cut food into smaller, bite-sized pieces, making them easier to chew and digest. Incorporate soft grains like quinoa or couscous, which are gentle on the digestive system. Additionally, avoid tough, fibrous foods like raw carrots, opting instead for cooked versions that are easier to manage.

Using Steaming and Roasting to Enhance Nutrient Absorption

Steaming is an excellent cooking method for enhancing nutrient absorption, as it preserves vitamins that are sensitive to heat and water. By gently steaming vegetables like spinach or broccoli, you retain their natural nutrients, especially vitamin C, which would otherwise be lost in boiling. Steaming also maintains the fiber content, which supports digestion and overall health. Pairing steamed vegetables with healthy fats, such as olive oil or avocado, further enhances the absorption of fat-soluble vitamins like A and K.

Roasting, on the other hand, adds flavor while preserving nutrients in foods like root vegetables and proteins. For instance, roasting carrots and sweet potatoes at moderate temperatures caramelizes their natural sugars without breaking down vitamins like beta-carotene. Drizzle olive oil over the vegetables before roasting to help the body better absorb these vitamins, making each meal more nutrient-dense and beneficial for lung health.

Chapter 14:

Meal Prep Tips for COPD Management

How to Plan and Prepare Meals in Advance for Convenience

To plan and prepare meals in advance for COPD, start by creating a weekly meal plan that includes nutrient-dense foods like leafy greens, lean proteins, and whole grains. Aim for a balance of vitamins, minerals, and healthy fats that support lung health and boost energy. Once you have your menu, make a shopping list based on the recipes. Choose simple recipes that can be prepared in bulk, ensuring each meal is packed with essential nutrients to manage symptoms and improve overall well-being.

When preparing meals, spend a few hours on a designated day (like Sunday) chopping vegetables, cooking proteins, and portioning meals into containers for easy access throughout the week. This will reduce stress during the busy workweek and help you stick to a healthy, COPD-friendly diet. Pre-cooking items like quinoa, brown rice, or roasted chicken allow for quick meal assembly, saving you time and ensuring you always have nutritious meals on hand.

Easy Meal Prep Ideas to Ensure a Nutrient-Rich Diet

An easy meal prep idea is to prepare a large salad using dark, leafy greens like spinach or kale, combined with antioxidant-rich vegetables such as bell peppers and tomatoes. Add lean proteins like grilled chicken or tofu, and drizzle with olive oil for healthy fats that help with inflammation. Portion these salads into containers so you can grab them quickly during the week. Another quick idea is to cook a batch of whole grains like quinoa or brown rice, which can be paired with a variety of proteins and vegetables for balanced meals.

For breakfasts, you can prepare overnight oats with oats, chia seeds, berries, and a splash of almond milk. This high-fiber, nutrient-packed meal can be made in advance, stored in the fridge, and eaten cold or warmed up. By planning a variety of easy meals, you'll maintain a nutrient-rich diet, ensuring your body gets the vitamins and minerals it needs to support lung function and energy levels.

Storing COPD-Friendly Meals for Quick Access throughout the Week

Once your meals are prepped, storing them properly ensures you can access them quickly throughout the week. Use clear, airtight containers to portion out meals into single servings, making it easier to grab and go. Store salads, cooked proteins, and grains separately to maintain freshness, and label containers with the date they were prepared. Keep quick snacks like sliced fruits, nuts, and yogurt in easy-to-reach areas of the fridge to ensure you always have COPD-friendly options on hand.

If you're prepping foods that need to last longer, consider refrigerating some meals for immediate consumption and freezing others for later in the week. For optimal freshness, meals stored in the refrigerator should be eaten within 3-4 days, while those in the freezer can last up to 2-3 months. Proper storage ensures that you'll always have a healthy meal ready, which reduces stress and helps you stay on track with your diet.

Batch Cooking Strategies to Save Time and Reduce Stress

Batch cooking is a fantastic strategy for saving time and ensuring you have healthy meals ready throughout the week. To start, pick a few COPD-friendly recipes, such as vegetable soups, stews, or casseroles that you can make in large quantities. Cook these meals in bulk, portion them into containers, and store them in the fridge or freezer. This reduces the daily burden of cooking and ensures you always have nutritious options available when you're tired or short on time.

Another effective batch cooking method is to prepare versatile base ingredients, like roasted vegetables, grilled chicken, or lentils, which can be mixed and matched with different sides for variety. For instance, roasted veggies can be added to salads, wraps, or grain bowls throughout the week. By batch cooking in advance, you'll not only save time but also ensure that healthy, balanced meals are always within reach.

COPD-Friendly Freezer Meal Ideas for Busy Days

Freezer meals are a lifesaver on busy days when you don't have time to cook but still want to eat healthy. COPD-friendly options include hearty vegetable soups, stews with lean meats, or casseroles made with whole grains and low-sodium ingredients. Simply portion these meals into freezer-safe containers after cooking, and freeze them for later use. To make it even easier, label each container with the date and reheating instructions, so you can quickly thaw and warm up your meals.

For an easy grab-and-go option, consider making breakfast burritos or egg muffins loaded with vegetables and lean protein. Freeze them individually, and on busy mornings, you can reheat them in the microwave for a quick, balanced meal. These freezer meals ensure that even on your busiest days, you have access to nutritious, lung-supportive food with minimal effort.

Chapter 15:

Common Dietary Concerns and Solutions

Managing Food-Related Fatigue and Shortness of Breath While Eating

To reduce fatigue and shortness of breath while eating, break meals into smaller, more frequent portions throughout the day. Instead of having three large meals, aim for five to six smaller meals that require less energy to eat. Soft, easy-to-chew foods like mashed potatoes, soups, or smoothies are beneficial because they require less effort, allowing for easier breathing and quicker digestion. Sitting upright during meals and eating slowly also helps prevent shortness of breath.

Another helpful approach is to conserve energy while preparing food by using pre-cut or pre-cooked ingredients. Choose nutrient-dense foods that pack more energy in smaller portions, like avocados, eggs, or nuts. Hydrate well but avoid drinking too much water during meals, as it can cause fullness and discomfort. Keeping meals simple and easy to manage can significantly reduce strain during eating.

How to Avoid Common Dietary Triggers for COPD Flare-Ups

Certain foods can exacerbate COPD symptoms, so it's important to avoid known dietary triggers. Foods that cause gas and bloating, like beans, carbonated beverages, and cruciferous vegetables (broccoli, cabbage), can increase pressure on the diaphragm, making breathing more difficult. Dairy products may also thicken mucus in some individuals, so it's worth limiting these if they worsen symptoms.

Additionally, high-sodium foods can lead to fluid retention, which may strain breathing. Stick to low-sodium alternatives and avoid processed or packaged foods that are often high in salt. Monitoring your diet for triggers and keeping a food diary can help you identify which items to avoid.

Tips for Improving Appetite and Ensuring Adequate Nutrition

Loss of appetite is common in COPD patients, but maintaining proper nutrition is essential for managing the disease. To stimulate your appetite, focus on foods that are visually appealing and easy to digest, such as colorful fruit salads or scrambled eggs. Incorporating small amounts of healthy fats, like olive oil or peanut butter, into your meals can increase calorie intake without overwhelming your stomach.

Snacking between meals can help, especially with nutrient-dense options like yogurt, nuts, or cheese. If eating solid food is difficult, try nutrient-rich smoothies or meal replacement shakes to ensure you're getting enough calories and vitamins.

Managing Food Intolerances and Allergies alongside COPD

Managing food intolerances and allergies with COPD requires careful planning. Start by identifying foods that trigger intolerances, such as dairy, gluten, or nuts, and find suitable alternatives that meet your nutritional needs. For instance, if dairy worsens your symptoms, switch to plant-based milks like almond or oat milk, which are often fortified with vitamins and calcium.

It's important to read food labels to avoid hidden allergens, and meal prep can help you stay in control of what you eat. Consult a nutritionist to ensure you're not missing out on key nutrients while managing both COPD and food sensitivities.

Strategies for Overcoming Common Cooking Challenges for COPD Patients

Cooking can be exhausting for COPD patients, but simplifying meal prep can make it more manageable. Focus on batch cooking or using appliances like slow cookers, which allow you to prepare large quantities of food with minimal effort. Pre-cut vegetables, canned beans, and ready-made sauces can reduce prep time and energy expenditure.

Consider sitting while chopping ingredients and use lightweight pots and pans to conserve energy. Organize your kitchen so commonly used items are within easy reach to avoid unnecessary movement. By breaking up tasks and focusing on convenience, cooking becomes less overwhelming and more sustainable.

Chapter 16:

Frequently Asked Questions (FAQs) About COPD Diet

What Foods Should Be Avoided for COPD Management?

For individuals managing COPD, avoiding foods that cause bloating or gas is crucial, as these can make breathing more difficult. Foods like carbonated beverages, fried or greasy meals, and certain vegetables such as broccoli, cabbage, and beans should be limited. These foods increase pressure on the diaphragm, making it harder for your lungs to expand. Processed foods high in salt are another concern, as excess sodium leads to water retention, increasing blood pressure and straining the heart and lungs.

Additionally, dairy products can sometimes thicken mucus, making it harder to clear airways. Replace whole milk with almond or oat milk alternatives, and opt for low-sodium, fresh foods over processed snacks. Pay attention to how your body reacts to specific foods and adjust accordingly to keep symptoms in check.

How Can I Get Enough Calories When I Feel Too Tired to Eat?

When you're fatigued from COPD, preparing and eating meals can feel overwhelming. To maintain proper calorie intake, opt for nutrient-dense, easy-to-prepare snacks and meals. Smoothies made with protein powder, fruits, and vegetables are quick to make and offer a calorie boost. Small, frequent meals are more manageable than large meals, so try eating every 2–3 hours rather than three large meals a day.

Another tip is to choose high-calorie, nutritious foods like nuts, seeds, avocados, and full-fat yogurt. Keep pre-cut vegetables, fruits, and ready-made healthy snacks on hand to avoid skipping meals. If cooking is too exhausting, consider meal prepping on better days or relying on healthy frozen meals to save energy.

Are There Any Supplements That Can Support Lung Health?

Several supplements may help support lung health in individuals with COPD. Omega-3 fatty acids, found in fish oil supplements, have anti-inflammatory properties that can aid in reducing lung inflammation. Antioxidants like vitamins C and E help combat oxidative stress, which can damage lung tissue. These can be taken as supplements or consumed through foods like citrus fruits and leafy greens.

Vitamin D is also essential, as deficiency has been linked to worsened lung function in COPD patients. Consider getting your vitamin D levels checked, and take a supplement if needed, especially during winter months. Always consult your healthcare provider before starting any new supplements to ensure they don't interact with your medications.

How Do I Manage Weight Loss or Gain With COPD?

Weight management is key for COPD patients, as both underweight and overweight conditions can worsen symptoms. If you're losing weight unintentionally, aim to increase your calorie intake with nutrient-dense, easy-to-eat foods like smoothies, nuts, and whole grains. Adding protein to every meal will help you maintain muscle mass, which is essential for respiratory strength.

For those gaining weight, particularly due to medications or inactivity, focus on portion control and balanced meals. Swap out refined carbs for whole grains and prioritize vegetables and lean proteins to maintain a healthy weight. Engaging in light physical activity, such as walking or seated exercises, can also help manage weight while improving lung function.

What Are the Best Beverages for Hydration and Lung Health?

Staying hydrated is essential for lung health, as it helps keep mucus thin and easier to expel. Water is the best choice, and you should aim for at least 6-8 glasses a day. Herbal teas like ginger or peppermint can also provide hydration while offering soothing effects for the airways. Avoid caffeinated drinks like coffee, which can lead to dehydration, and limit alcohol, which can interact with medications.

If plain water is unappealing, try adding slices of citrus, cucumber, or berries for natural flavor. Low-sodium broths can also be hydrating and comforting, particularly on colder days or when you're not feeling well. Make hydration a priority, as it directly impacts how well your lungs function.

Chapter 17:

Supplements and COPD: What You Need to Know

Key Vitamins and Minerals That Support Respiratory Health

Vitamins and minerals play a crucial role in maintaining lung health and managing COPD symptoms. Vitamin C, for example, acts as an antioxidant, reducing inflammation in the airways and boosting immune function, while Vitamin D strengthens the immune system and helps reduce respiratory infections. Magnesium is also essential, as it relaxes the muscles around the airways, making breathing easier. Including foods rich in these nutrients, such as citrus fruits, leafy greens, and fish, can significantly support lung function.

Additionally, Vitamin E and omega-3 fatty acids found in nuts, seeds, and fish help reduce oxidative stress in the lungs. Zinc is another important mineral that helps the body fight off infections, which is vital for those with COPD. Incorporating these key vitamins and minerals through whole foods can boost lung capacity and help manage symptoms more effectively.

Best Supplements for Improving Lung Function and Reducing Symptoms

Certain supplements can effectively enhance lung function and reduce COPD symptoms. Omega-3 fatty acids, commonly found in fish oil supplements, have been shown to reduce airway inflammation, improving breathing and lung capacity. Another beneficial supplement is N-acetylcysteine (NAC), which helps break down mucus in the lungs, making it easier to expel and reducing congestion.

Vitamin D supplements are also valuable for those with COPD, especially in individuals with a deficiency, as they can reduce exacerbations and improve overall lung health. Consult a healthcare professional to determine the right dosage and combination of these supplements for your specific needs.

How to Choose COPD-Friendly Supplements

When choosing supplements for COPD, it's essential to focus on those that improve lung function and boost immunity without causing side effects. Look for high-quality, third-party-tested supplements that contain essential nutrients like Omega-3 fatty acids, Vitamin D, and magnesium. Supplements should be free from fillers and additives that could trigger respiratory issues, so always check the label for purity.

Consulting with a healthcare provider before starting new supplements is vital, especially for COPD patients, as interactions with medications can occur. Opt for supplements in forms that are easy to digest, such as capsules or liquid, to prevent any digestive discomfort that could worsen symptoms.

Understanding the Role of Probiotics in COPD Management

Probiotics, beneficial bacteria found in the gut, can play a significant role in managing COPD by supporting the immune system and reducing inflammation. Research suggests that a healthy gut microbiome helps regulate the body's response to infections and inflammation, both of which are key factors in COPD. Probiotics can be found in foods like yogurt, kefir, and sauerkraut or taken as a supplement.

Introducing probiotics into your diet can improve lung function by reducing harmful bacteria in the respiratory tract. Maintaining gut health with regular intake of probiotics may lower the frequency and severity of COPD flare-ups, making it a valuable addition to your overall management strategy.

When to Consider Adding Supplements to Your Diet

It's essential to consider adding supplements to your diet if you are not getting enough nutrients from food alone, especially if you have COPD. If you experience frequent respiratory infections, fatigue, or difficulty managing symptoms, supplements like Vitamin D, Omega-3 fatty acids, and N-acetylcysteine (NAC) may help. Regular blood tests can identify deficiencies, and your doctor may recommend specific supplements to address these.

Begin incorporating supplements gradually, ensuring you monitor any changes in symptoms. Adding supplements can be particularly beneficial during colder months when respiratory infections are more common, or when dietary intake of key nutrients is reduced. Always consult a healthcare provider before starting any new supplement regimen.

Chapter 18:

Dining Out with COPD: Making Healthy Choices

How to Navigate Restaurant Menus with COPD in Mind

When dining out with COPD, focus on selecting nutrient-dense foods that support lung health. Look for dishes rich in fruits, vegetables, lean proteins, and whole grains. Avoid fried or highly processed options, as they often contain added sodium and unhealthy fats. Opt for steamed, grilled, or baked preparations, and ask for dressings and sauces on the side to control sodium intake.

Reading the menu carefully can also help. Many restaurants have healthier sections or customizable meals. Choose smaller portions or split an entrée with a friend to prevent overeating, which can affect breathing. Be mindful of ingredients like excess dairy, which can increase mucus production.

Tips for Choosing Low-Sodium, Lung-Friendly Options When Dining Out

When eating out, always prioritize low-sodium options to avoid worsening COPD symptoms. Request unsalted, grilled meats, or fish as your main dish, and choose steamed vegetables or salads as sides. Skip dishes labeled "smoked," "cured," or "fried," as they are usually high in sodium.

You can also ask for your meal to be prepared without added salt or request oil-based dressings instead of creamy sauces. Focus on fresh, whole foods and avoid breaded or processed ingredients that can negatively impact your lung health.

How to Communicate Dietary Needs to Restaurant Staff

When dining out, don't hesitate to communicate your dietary needs clearly to the staff. Politely ask questions about the preparation of dishes and inquire if modifications are possible, such as removing added salt, using olive oil instead of butter, or grilling instead of frying. Most restaurants are willing to accommodate dietary restrictions when explained courteously.

Consider explaining your condition briefly and emphasizing the importance of lower sodium and healthier preparation methods. Asking for allergen-free or diet-specific menus can also make the selection process smoother. Practicing clear communication ensures that your meal aligns with your COPD needs.

Managing Portion Sizes and Avoiding Overeating in Social Settings

To avoid overeating, especially when dining out or in social gatherings, consider starting with a smaller portion. Many restaurants offer large servings, which can cause discomfort and make it harder to breathe. You can always take half of your meal home or share it with someone to avoid overconsumption.

Another helpful strategy is to eat slowly and listen to your body's cues of fullness. Drinking water between bites can help with digestion and portion control. Social settings may encourage larger portions, but mindful eating and choosing healthier options will help manage COPD symptoms more effectively.

Healthy Snack Ideas to Bring When Traveling or Dining Out

When traveling or dining out, it's helpful to carry healthy, lung-friendly snacks. Pack options like unsalted nuts, sliced fruits, whole-grain crackers, or raw vegetables. These snacks are nutrient-dense and low in sodium, making them ideal for COPD management on the go.

Preparing homemade snacks, such as low-sodium hummus with veggie sticks or air-popped popcorn, can keep you on track when eating out. By bringing your snacks, you'll have better control over your diet and avoid high-sodium or unhealthy processed snacks often found when traveling or at restaurants.

Chapter 19:

Creating a Long-Term COPD Diet Plan

How to Develop a Personalized COPD-Friendly Meal Plan

Creating a personalized meal plan for COPD involves focusing on nutrient-dense foods that support lung health and overall well-being. Start by incorporating a variety of fruits, vegetables, whole grains, and lean proteins into your diet. Foods rich in antioxidants, such as berries and leafy greens, can help reduce inflammation and support lung function. Additionally, consider including sources of omega-3 fatty acids like fatty fish, which may help in reducing respiratory symptoms.

When planning meals, ensure they are balanced and cater to your specific symptoms and preferences. It's helpful to consult with a dietitian who can tailor the meal plan based on your individual health needs and any dietary restrictions. For example, if you experience breathlessness, eating smaller, more frequent meals may prevent discomfort. Document your food intake and monitor how different foods affect your symptoms to make necessary adjustments.

Adjusting Your Diet Based on Symptom Changes and Flare-Ups

Adjusting your diet in response to symptom changes involves paying close attention to how different foods impact your COPD. During flare-ups, focus on consuming soft, easily digestible foods that are low in sodium to avoid fluid retention. For instance, you might switch to mashed potatoes, steamed vegetables, or soups instead of raw, fibrous foods that could exacerbate coughing or shortness of breath.

Keep a food diary to track your symptoms and identify any patterns related to your diet. If you notice specific foods worsening your symptoms, such as dairy or highly processed foods, it may be beneficial to eliminate or reduce these from your diet. Regular consultations with a healthcare provider can help you refine your diet based on ongoing symptom evaluation.

Tips for Maintaining a Balanced Diet During Busy or Stressful Times

Maintaining a balanced diet during hectic periods can be challenging, but with some strategic planning, it's achievable. Prepare and store healthy meals in advance to ensure you have nutritious options available even when you're busy. Utilize meal prep techniques like batch cooking and freezing portions of meals to simplify your eating routine.

When under stress, prioritize quick, easy-to-make dishes that are still healthy. For example, keep pre-chopped vegetables and whole grain wraps on hand for a fast, nutrient-packed meal. Opt for snacks like nuts, yogurt, and fruit to maintain energy levels without needing elaborate preparation.

Strategies for Staying Consistent with Meal Prep and Healthy Eating

Consistency in meal prep and healthy eating can be achieved through organization and habit formation. Create a weekly meal plan and shopping list to streamline grocery shopping and cooking. Dedicate specific times each week for meal preparation to avoid last-minute unhealthy food choices.

Consider using tools like meal prep containers to portion out meals and make them easily accessible. Set reminders for meal times and use apps to track your dietary intake, which can help keep you accountable and focused on your nutritional goals.

Long-Term Nutritional Goals to Support Optimal Respiratory Wellness

Long-term nutritional goals for supporting respiratory wellness involve sustaining a diet that continually promotes lung health and overall vitality. Aim for a balanced intake of vitamins and minerals essential for respiratory function, such as vitamin C, vitamin D, and magnesium.

Incorporate a variety of foods to ensure a comprehensive nutrient profile.

Regularly review and adjust your diet to meet evolving health needs and lifestyle changes. For example, as you age or if your COPD symptoms change, you might need to increase your intake of certain nutrients or adjust your meal frequency. Regular follow-ups with a healthcare provider can help ensure your diet remains aligned with your long-term health goals.

21 Days Meal Plan Recipes plus Ingredients and their Preparations

DAY 1: Grilled Salmon with Quinoa and Kale Salad

Ingredients:

- 1 salmon fillet (5-6 oz)
- ½ cup quinoa
- 1 cup kale, chopped
- ½ lemon, juiced
- 1 tbsp olive oil
- Salt and pepper to taste
- 1 clove garlic, minced

Preparation:

- Preheat the grill to medium heat. Season the salmon with olive oil, salt, and pepper.

- Cook the quinoa according to package instructions, then set aside.

- Grill the salmon for 4-5 minutes on each side until fully cooked.

- In a large bowl, toss the chopped kale with lemon juice, olive oil, garlic, salt, and pepper.

- Serve the grilled salmon over the quinoa, with a kale salad on the side.

DAY 2: Baked Chicken with Sweet Potatoes and Spinach

Ingredients:

- 1 chicken breast (boneless, skinless)

- 1 medium sweet potato, peeled and cubed
- 1 cup fresh spinach
- 1 tbsp olive oil

- 1 tsp paprika
- Salt and pepper to taste

Preparation:

- Preheat the oven to 375°F (190°C). Season the chicken breast with olive oil, paprika, salt, and pepper.
- Place the sweet potatoes on a baking sheet, drizzle with olive oil, and season with salt and pepper.
- Bake the chicken and sweet potatoes for 25-30 minutes until the chicken is fully cooked and the sweet potatoes are tender.
- Sauté the spinach in a pan with a little olive oil and salt for 2-3 minutes.
- Serve the chicken with baked sweet potatoes and sautéed spinach.

DAY 3: Lentil and Vegetable Stew

Ingredients:

- 1 cup green lentils
- 1 carrot, chopped
- 1 celery stalk, chopped
- ½ onion, diced
- 1 zucchini, chopped
- 2 garlic cloves, minced
- 1 tbsp olive oil
- 4 cups low-sodium vegetable broth
- 1 tsp turmeric
- 1 tsp cumin
- Salt and pepper to taste

Preparation:

- Heat the olive oil in a large pot over medium heat. Add the onion, garlic, carrot, and celery. Cook for 5-7 minutes.
- Add the lentils, vegetable

broth, turmeric, cumin, salt, and pepper.

- Bring to a boil, then reduce the heat and simmer for 25-30 minutes.

- Add the zucchini in the last 10 minutes of cooking.

- Serve the lentil stew warm.

DAY 4: Turkey and Avocado Lettuce Wraps

Ingredients:

- 4 large lettuce leaves (romaine or butter lettuce)
- 4 oz ground turkey
- ½ avocado, sliced
- 1 small cucumber, sliced
- 1 tbsp olive oil
- 1 tsp cumin
- 1 tsp chili powder
- Salt and pepper to taste

Preparation:

- Heat the olive oil in a pan over medium heat. Add the ground turkey, cumin, chili powder, salt, and pepper. Cook until the turkey is browned and fully cooked.

- Lay the lettuce leaves flat and place a portion of the cooked turkey in the center of each leaf.

- Top with avocado and cucumber slices.

- Roll the lettuce wraps and serve.

DAY 5: Shrimp Stir-Fry with Brown Rice

Ingredients:

- 6 oz shrimp, peeled and deveined
- 1 cup broccoli florets

- ½ red bell pepper, sliced
- 1 small carrot, julienned
- 2 tbsp low-sodium soy sauce

- 1 tbsp sesame oil
- 1 tsp ginger, minced
- 1 clove garlic, minced
- ½ cup cooked brown rice

Preparation:

- Heat sesame oil in a pan over medium-high heat. Add garlic and ginger, and sauté for 1 minute.

- Add the shrimp and cook for 3-4 minutes until pink.
- Toss in the broccoli, bell pepper, and carrot. Stir-fry for 5-7 minutes.
- Drizzle with soy sauce and serve over cooked brown rice.

DAY 6: Grilled Chicken and Asparagus with Almonds

Ingredients:

- 1 chicken breast (boneless, skinless)
- 8-10 asparagus spears
- 1 tbsp olive oil
- 1 tbsp slivered almonds
- ½ lemon, juiced
- Salt and pepper to taste

Preparation:

- Preheat the grill to medium heat. Season the chicken breast with olive oil, salt, and pepper.

- Grill the chicken for 5-7 minutes on each side until fully cooked.
- While the chicken grills, toss the asparagus in olive oil, salt, and pepper, and grill for 4-5 minutes until tender.
- Toast the almonds in a dry pan until golden.
- Drizzle the chicken and asparagus with lemon juice and sprinkle with almonds before serving.

DAY 7: Baked Cod with Roasted Brussels Sprouts

Ingredients:

- 1 cod fillet (5-6 oz)
- 1 cup Brussels sprouts, halved
- 1 tbsp olive oil
- ½ lemon, juiced
- 1 clove garlic, minced
- Salt and pepper to taste

Preparation:

- Preheat the oven to 400°F (200°C). Place the Brussels sprouts on a baking sheet, drizzle with olive oil, and season with salt and pepper. Roast for 20-25 minutes.
- Season the cod fillet with olive oil, garlic, lemon juice, salt, and pepper.
- Bake the cod for 12-15 minutes, or until the fish is opaque and flakes easily with a fork.
- Serve the baked cod with roasted Brussels sprouts.

DAY 8: Quinoa-Stuffed Bell Peppers

Ingredients:

- 2 large bell peppers
- ½ cup cooked quinoa
- ¼ cup black beans (canned, drained, and rinsed)
- ¼ cup corn kernels
- 1 small tomato, diced
- 1 tsp cumin
- 1 tbsp olive oil
- Salt and pepper to taste

Preparation:

- Preheat the oven to 375°F (190°C). Cut the tops off the bell peppers and remove the seeds.
- In a bowl, mix cooked quinoa, black beans, corn, tomato, cumin, olive oil, salt, and pepper.
- Stuff the bell peppers with the quinoa mixture and

place them in a baking dish.

- Bake for 20-25 minutes until the peppers are tender.
- Serve warm.

DAY 9: Tilapia with Garlic Mashed Cauliflower

Ingredients:

- 1 tilapia fillet (5-6 oz)
- 1 small head of cauliflower, chopped
- 1 clove garlic, minced
- 1 tbsp olive oil
- 1 tbsp fresh parsley, chopped
- Salt and pepper to taste

Preparation:

- Steam the cauliflower until tender, about 10-12 minutes.

- In a bowl, mash the cauliflower with garlic, olive oil, salt, and pepper.
- Heat a pan with a little olive oil and cook the tilapia for 3-4 minutes on each side until cooked through.
- Serve the tilapia with mashed cauliflower and sprinkle with fresh parsley.

DAY 10: Beef and Broccoli Stir-Fry

Ingredients:

- 4 oz lean beef strips
- 1 cup broccoli florets
- ½ onion, sliced

- 1 tbsp low-sodium soy sauce
- 1 tbsp sesame oil
- 1 tsp ginger, minced
- Salt and pepper to taste

Preparation:

- Heat sesame oil in a pan over medium-high heat. Add ginger and beef strips, and stir-fry for 4-5 minutes until browned.

- Add the broccoli and onion, and stir-fry for another 5-7 minutes.
- Drizzle with soy sauce and cook for an additional 2 minutes.
- Serve warm.

DAY 11: Chicken and Avocado Salad

Ingredients:

- 1 chicken breast (grilled)
- ½ avocado, sliced
- 1 cup mixed greens (spinach, arugula)
- 1 small cucumber, sliced
- 1 tbsp olive oil
- ½ lemon, juiced
- Salt and pepper to taste

Preparation:

- Grill the chicken breast and slice it into strips.
- In a bowl, combine mixed greens, avocado, and cucumber.
- Top with grilled chicken and drizzle with olive oil and lemon juice.
- Season with salt and pepper and toss the salad before serving.

DAY 12: Baked Trout with Steamed Green Beans

Ingredients:

- 1 trout fillet (5-6 oz)
- 1 cup green beans, trimmed
- 1 tbsp olive oil

- 1 tsp lemon zest
- 1 clove garlic, minced
- Salt and pepper to taste

Preparation:

- Preheat the oven to 375°F (190°C). Season the trout with olive oil, garlic, lemon zest, salt, and pepper.
- Bake the trout for 12-15 minutes, or until the fish is flaky.
- Steam the green beans for 5-7 minutes until tender.
- Serve the baked trout with steamed green beans.

DAY 13: Turkey and Vegetable Skillet

Ingredients:

- 4 oz ground turkey
- 1 cup bell peppers, chopped
- ½ cup zucchini, sliced
- ½ cup cherry tomatoes, halved
- 1 tbsp olive oil
- 1 tsp Italian seasoning
- Salt and pepper to taste

Preparation:

- Heat olive oil in a skillet over medium heat. Add ground turkey and cook until browned.
- Add bell peppers, zucchini, and cherry tomatoes. Cook for 5-7 minutes until vegetables are tender.
- Season with Italian seasoning, salt, and pepper.
- Serve warm.

DAY 14: Salmon and Spinach Frittata

- **Ingredients:**
- 2 eggs
- 2 oz smoked salmon, flaked
- 1 cup fresh spinach
- 1 tbsp olive oil
- Salt and pepper to taste

Preparation:

- Preheat the oven to 375°F (190°C). Heat olive oil in an oven-safe skillet over medium heat.
- Add spinach and cook until wilted.
- In a bowl, whisk eggs, salt, and pepper. Pour over the spinach into the skillet.

DAY 15: Greek Chicken Salad

Ingredients:

- 1 chicken breast (grilled, sliced)
- 1 cup cherry tomatoes, halved
- ½ cucumber, sliced
- ¼ cup Kalamata olives
- ¼ cup crumbled feta cheese
- 1 tbsp olive oil
- 1 tbsp red wine vinegar
- 1 tsp dried oregano
- Salt and pepper to taste

Preparation:

- Add smoked salmon on top and cook on the stove for 2 minutes.
- Transfer the skillet to the oven and bake for 10-12 minutes until the frittata is set.
- Serve warm.

- In a large bowl, combine cherry tomatoes, cucumber, olives, and feta cheese.
- Add the sliced grilled chicken.
- In a small bowl, whisk together olive oil, red wine vinegar, oregano, salt, and pepper.
- Drizzle the dressing over the salad and toss to combine.
- Serve immediately.

DAY 16: Chicken and Butternut Squash Bake

Ingredients:

- 1 chicken breast (boneless, skinless)
- 1 cup butternut squash, peeled and cubed
- 1 tbsp olive oil
- 1 tsp rosemary
- 1 clove garlic, minced
- Salt and pepper to taste

Preparation:

- Preheat the oven to 375°F (190°C). Season the chicken breast with olive oil, rosemary, garlic, salt, and pepper.
- Place the butternut squash on a baking sheet, drizzle with olive oil, and season with salt and pepper.
- Bake the chicken and butternut squash for 25-30 minutes, or until the chicken is cooked through and the squash is tender.
- Serve warm.

DAY 17: Spaghetti Squash with Tomato Basil Sauce

Ingredients:

- 1 small spaghetti squash
- 1 cup tomato sauce (low-sodium)
- 1 tsp dried basil
- 1 tbsp olive oil
- 1 clove garlic, minced
- Salt and pepper to taste

Preparation:

- Preheat the oven to 400°F (200°C). Cut the spaghetti squash in half and remove the seeds.
- Place the squash cut-side down on a baking sheet and bake for 40-45 minutes, or until tender.
- While the squash bakes,

heat olive oil in a pan and sauté garlic until fragrant.

- Add tomato sauce, dried basil, salt, and pepper. Simmer for 5 minutes.

- Once the squash is done, scrape the flesh with a fork to create "spaghetti."

- Top with the tomato basil sauce and serve.

DAY 18: Cod with Lemon and Herbs

Ingredients:

- 1 cod fillet (5-6 oz)
- 1 lemon, sliced
- 1 tbsp fresh parsley, chopped
- 1 tbsp olive oil
- Salt and pepper to taste

Preparation:

- Preheat the oven to 375°F (190°C). Place the cod fillet on a baking sheet.
- Drizzle with olive oil and season with salt and pepper.
- Top with lemon slices and chopped parsley.
- Bake for 12-15 minutes, or until the cod is opaque and flakes easily with a fork.
- Serve warm.

DAY 19: Sweet Potato and Black Bean Bowl

Ingredients:

- 1 medium sweet potato, peeled and cubed
- ½ cup black beans (canned, drained, and rinsed)
- 1 avocado, sliced
- 1 cup baby spinach
- 1 tbsp olive oil
- 1 tsp cumin
- Salt and pepper to taste

Preparation:

- Preheat the oven to 400°F (200°C). Toss sweet potato cubes with olive oil, cumin, salt, and pepper.
- Roast sweet potatoes for 25-30 minutes until tender.
- In a bowl, combine roasted sweet potatoes, black beans, avocado slices, and baby spinach.
- Serve immediately.

DAY 20: Chicken and Vegetable Stir-Fry

Ingredients:

- 1 chicken breast, sliced
- 1 cup bell peppers, sliced
- ½ cup snap peas
- ½ cup carrots, sliced
- 1 tbsp olive oil
- 2 tbsp low-sodium soy sauce
- 1 tsp ginger, minced
- Salt and pepper to taste

Preparation:

- Heat olive oil in a pan over medium-high heat. Add chicken and cook until browned and cooked through.
- Add bell peppers, snap peas, and carrots. Stir-fry for 5-7 minutes until vegetables are tender.
- Drizzle with soy sauce and add ginger. Cook for an additional 2 minutes.
- Serve warm.

DAY 21: Vegetable and Hummus Wrap

Ingredients:

- 1 whole wheat tortilla
- 2 tbsp hummus
- ¼ cup shredded carrots
- ¼ cup sliced bell peppers
- ¼ cup cucumber, sliced
- ¼ cup baby spinach
- Salt and pepper to taste

Preparation:

- Spread hummus evenly over the whole wheat tortilla.
- Layer with shredded carrots, bell peppers, cucumber, and baby spinach.
- Season with salt and pepper.
- Roll up the tortilla and slice it in half.
- Serve immediately.

Author's appreciation

Thank you for exploring "The COPD Diet Cookbook: Nutrient-Rich Recipes to Improve Lung Health, Boost Energy, and Manage Symptoms for Optimal Respiratory Wellness." We hope these meal plans and recipes provide you with delicious, nourishing options that support your respiratory health and overall well-being.

Your commitment to managing COPD through thoughtful dietary choices is commendable. Each recipe in this book is crafted with care to offer you the best in flavor and nutrition while helping to alleviate symptoms and enhance your quality of life.

Remember, every meal is an opportunity to nurture your body and embrace a healthier lifestyle. We appreciate your dedication to this journey and wish you continued success in your efforts to breathe easier and live well.

Made in the USA
Columbia, SC
06 February 2025

53420288R00061